THE ULTIMATE DIABETIC DIET COOKBOOK AFTER 50

A Beginner's Guide To 2000+ Days Of Nourishing And Tasty Low-Carb, Low-Sugar & Low-Fat Recipes For Newly Diagnosed, Type 1 & 2 Diabetes, With A 31-Day Meal Plan

Angelo Melvin

Table of Contents

COPYRIGHT © 2023

CHAPTER ONE

Understanding Diabetes and Nutrition

Diabetes is a complex metabolic disorder characterized by high blood sugar levels over a prolonged period. It occurs when the pancreas does not produce enough insulin or when the body cannot effectively use the insulin it produces. Proper nutrition plays a crucial role in managing diabetes, as it helps regulate blood sugar levels and reduce the risk of complications. In this comprehensive guide, we'll delve into the intricacies of diabetes and its relationship with nutrition.

What is Diabetes?

Diabetes mellitus, commonly referred to as diabetes, is a chronic medical condition that affects how your body metabolizes glucose, the main source of energy. Glucose is derived from the foods we consume and is transported into the cells with the help of insulin, a hormone produced by the pancreas. In diabetes, there are two primary abnormalities: inadequate insulin production by the pancreas or ineffective utilization of insulin by the body's cells, leading to elevated blood sugar levels.

There are three main types of diabetes:

1. **Type 1 Diabetes**: This type of diabetes occurs when the immune system mistakenly attacks and destroys the insulin-producing beta cells in the pancreas. As a result, the body

cannot produce enough insulin to regulate blood sugar levels. Type 1 diabetes is typically diagnosed in children and young adults, although it can develop at any age. Management of type 1 diabetes involves daily insulin injections or the use of an insulin pump, along with careful monitoring of blood sugar levels and dietary intake.

2. **Type 2 Diabetes**: Type 2 diabetes is the most common form of diabetes, accounting for approximately 90% of all cases. It develops when the body becomes resistant to the effects of insulin or when the pancreas fails to produce enough insulin to meet the body's needs. Type 2 diabetes is often associated with obesity, sedentary lifestyle, and genetic predisposition. Unlike type 1 diabetes, type 2 diabetes can sometimes be managed through lifestyle modifications, including diet, exercise, and weight loss, although medications or insulin therapy may also be necessary.

3. **Gestational Diabetes**: Gestational diabetes occurs during pregnancy and is characterized by high blood sugar levels that develop or are first recognized during pregnancy. It can increase the risk of complications for both the mother and the baby, including preeclampsia, macrosomia (large birth weight), and the need for cesarean delivery. While gestational diabetes usually resolves after childbirth, women

who have had gestational diabetes are at increased risk of developing type 2 diabetes later in life.

Types of Diabetes After 50

As individuals age, their risk of developing diabetes increases due to various factors, including changes in metabolism, decreased physical activity, and changes in body composition. After the age of 50, the prevalence of diabetes tends to rise, particularly type 2 diabetes. This age-related increase in diabetes risk is attributed to a combination of genetic predisposition, lifestyle factors, and age-related physiological changes.

In addition to type 2 diabetes, older adults may also be at risk of developing other forms of diabetes, such as latent autoimmune diabetes in adults (LADA) and maturity-onset diabetes of the young (MODY). LADA shares features of both type 1 and type 2 diabetes and is characterized by the gradual onset of autoimmune destruction of pancreatic beta cells in adults. MODY is a rare form of diabetes that is inherited and typically presents before the age of 25, although it can sometimes go undiagnosed until later in life.

Managing diabetes after the age of 50 requires a comprehensive approach that takes into account the individual's health status, lifestyle habits, and nutritional needs. Older adults with diabetes may have unique dietary requirements and may benefit from dietary modifications to optimize blood sugar control, prevent complications, and promote overall health and well-being.

The Role of Diet in Managing Diabetes

Diet plays a central role in the management of diabetes, as it directly influences blood sugar levels, insulin sensitivity, and overall health. A well-balanced diet can help individuals with diabetes achieve and maintain optimal blood sugar control, prevent complications, and improve quality of life. Several dietary strategies are recommended for managing diabetes:

1. **Carbohydrate Counting**: Carbohydrate counting is a meal-planning approach that involves tracking the amount of carbohydrates consumed at each meal and matching it with the appropriate dose of insulin or other diabetes medications. Carbohydrates have the most significant impact on blood sugar levels, so monitoring carbohydrate intake is crucial for managing blood sugar levels in individuals with diabetes.

2. **Glycemic Index**: The glycemic index (GI) is a measure of how quickly a carbohydrate-containing food raises blood sugar levels. Foods with a low GI are digested and absorbed more slowly, resulting in a gradual rise in blood sugar levels, whereas foods with a high GI cause a rapid increase in blood sugar levels. Choosing foods with a lower GI can help

stabilize blood sugar levels and improve glycemic control in individuals with diabetes.

3. **Fiber-Rich Foods**: Fiber is an essential nutrient that plays a key role in managing diabetes. It helps slow down the absorption of sugar into the bloodstream, which can help prevent spikes in blood sugar levels after meals. Additionally, fiber helps promote satiety, regulate bowel movements, and improve cholesterol levels. Incorporating fiber-rich foods such as fruits, vegetables, whole grains, legumes, and nuts into the diet can help individuals with diabetes achieve better blood sugar control and overall health.

4. **Healthy Fats**: Healthy fats, such as monounsaturated and polyunsaturated fats found in nuts, seeds, avocados, and fatty fish, can help improve insulin sensitivity and reduce the risk of cardiovascular disease in individuals with diabetes. Including sources of healthy fats in the diet can help balance blood sugar levels, promote satiety, and support heart health.

5. **Portion Control**: Controlling portion sizes is essential for managing diabetes, as overeating can lead to spikes in blood sugar levels. Using smaller plates, measuring portions, and being mindful of portion sizes can help individuals with diabetes avoid overconsumption and maintain better blood sugar control.

6. **Regular Meal Timing**: Eating meals and snacks at regular intervals throughout the day can help stabilize blood sugar levels and prevent fluctuations. Skipping meals or going for long periods without eating can lead to drops in blood sugar levels and increase the risk of overeating later on. Aim to eat meals and snacks at consistent times each day to maintain steady energy levels and support blood sugar control.

7. **Hydration**: Staying hydrated is important for overall health and can also help manage diabetes. Drinking an adequate amount of water can help prevent dehydration, support kidney function, and regulate blood sugar levels. Aim to drink plenty of water throughout the day and limit intake of sugary beverages such as soda, fruit juice, and sweetened teas.

In addition to these dietary strategies, it's essential for individuals with diabetes to work closely with a healthcare provider or registered dietitian to develop a personalized meal plan that meets their nutritional needs, preferences, and health goals. Regular monitoring of blood sugar levels, along with adjustments to diet and medication as needed, can help individuals with diabetes achieve optimal glycemic control and improve their overall quality of life. By adopting a healthy and balanced diet, individuals with diabetes can effectively manage their condition and reduce the risk of complications, allowing them to lead full and active lives.

CHAPTER TWO

Essentials of a Diabetic Diet

A diabetic diet is a crucial component of managing diabetes effectively. It focuses on controlling blood sugar levels, promoting overall health, and reducing the risk of complications associated with diabetes. By making informed food choices and adopting healthy eating habits, individuals with diabetes can better manage their condition and improve their quality of life. In this section, we'll explore the essentials of a diabetic diet, including the balance of macronutrients, the importance of fiber and whole grains, and strategies for managing portion sizes and meal timing.

Balancing Carbohydrates, Proteins, and Fats

Balancing carbohydrates, proteins, and fats is fundamental to maintaining stable blood sugar levels and managing diabetes. Each macronutrient plays a unique role in the body and has a different effect on blood sugar levels:

1. **Carbohydrates**: Carbohydrates have the most significant impact on blood sugar levels as they are broken down into glucose during digestion. Therefore, it's essential for individuals with diabetes to monitor their carbohydrate intake and choose carbohydrates wisely. Focus on consuming complex carbohydrates, such as whole grains, legumes, fruits, and vegetables, which are digested more slowly and have a less dramatic effect on blood sugar levels

compared to simple carbohydrates like refined grains and sugars.

2. **Proteins**: Protein is essential for building and repairing tissues, maintaining muscle mass, and supporting overall health. While protein does not directly affect blood sugar levels, it can impact insulin sensitivity and satiety. Including lean sources of protein such as poultry, fish, tofu, beans, and lentils in meals and snacks can help stabilize blood sugar levels and promote feelings of fullness.

3. **Fats**: Healthy fats, such as monounsaturated and polyunsaturated fats, play a crucial role in managing diabetes and supporting heart health. Unlike carbohydrates, fats have minimal impact on blood sugar levels and can help slow down the absorption of carbohydrates, leading to more stable blood sugar levels. Sources of healthy fats include nuts, seeds, avocado, olive oil, and fatty fish like salmon and mackerel.

Achieving a balance of carbohydrates, proteins, and fats in each meal and snack can help individuals with diabetes optimize blood sugar control, promote satiety, and support overall health and well-being.

Importance of Fiber and Whole Grains

Fiber is a type of carbohydrate found in plant foods that the body cannot digest or absorb. It plays a crucial role in managing diabetes by slowing down the absorption of sugar into the bloodstream, promoting satiety, and improving digestive health. Incorporating fiber-rich foods into the diet can help individuals with diabetes achieve better blood sugar control and reduce the risk of complications. Some sources of dietary fiber include:

- **Whole Grains**: Whole grains, such as brown rice, quinoa, barley, oats, and whole wheat, are rich in fiber, vitamins, minerals, and antioxidants. They provide sustained energy and help stabilize blood sugar levels, making them an excellent choice for individuals with diabetes.

- **Fruits and Vegetables**: Fruits and vegetables are naturally low in calories and rich in fiber, vitamins, and minerals. They can help satisfy hunger, control cravings, and improve blood sugar control when consumed as part of a balanced diet.

- **Legumes**: Legumes, including beans, lentils, chickpeas, and peas, are high in fiber and protein and have a low glycemic index, making them an excellent choice for individuals with diabetes. They can help regulate blood sugar levels, promote fullness, and support heart health.

- **Nuts and Seeds**: Nuts and seeds are rich in fiber, healthy fats, protein, and other nutrients. They make a convenient and nutritious snack option for individuals with diabetes and can help stabilize blood sugar levels when consumed in moderation.

Incorporating fiber-rich foods such as whole grains, fruits, vegetables, legumes, nuts, and seeds into meals and snacks can help individuals with diabetes improve glycemic control, promote satiety, and support overall health and well-being.

Managing Portion Sizes and Meal Timing

Managing portion sizes and meal timing is essential for controlling blood sugar levels and preventing spikes and dips throughout the day. Here are some strategies for managing portion sizes and meal timing:

1. **Use Portion Control Tools**: Use measuring cups, spoons, and food scales to accurately measure portion sizes and avoid overeating. Pay attention to serving sizes listed on food labels and aim to consume appropriate portions to prevent excess calorie intake and maintain blood sugar control.

2. **Fill Half Your Plate with Non-Starchy Vegetables**: Non-starchy vegetables such as leafy greens, broccoli, cauliflower, peppers, and cucumbers are low in calories and carbohydrates and high in fiber, vitamins, and minerals. By filling half your plate with non-starchy vegetables, you can increase your fiber intake, promote satiety, and control blood sugar levels.

3. **Eat Regularly Scheduled Meals and Snacks**: Eating meals and snacks at regular intervals throughout the day can help stabilize blood sugar levels and prevent fluctuations. Aim to

eat breakfast, lunch, dinner, and snacks at consistent times each day to maintain steady energy levels and support blood sugar control.

4. **Be Mindful of Portion Sizes of Carbohydrates**: While carbohydrates are an essential part of a balanced diet, it's crucial to be mindful of portion sizes, especially if you have diabetes. Aim to include a moderate amount of carbohydrates in each meal and snack, and choose carbohydrates that are high in fiber and low in added sugars to help regulate blood sugar levels.

5. **Practice Mindful Eating**: Pay attention to hunger and fullness cues, and eat slowly and mindfully to prevent overeating. Focus on enjoying your food and savoring each bite, and stop eating when you feel satisfied rather than overly full.

By practicing portion control, choosing nutrient-dense foods, and eating meals and snacks at regular intervals, individuals with diabetes can better manage their blood sugar levels, promote satiety, and support overall health and well-being. Working with a healthcare provider or registered dietitian can help develop a personalized meal plan that meets individual nutritional needs, preferences, and health goals.

CHAPTER THREE

Meal Planning and Preparation Tips

Meal planning and preparation are essential components of managing diabetes effectively. By creating balanced meal plans, making smart grocery shopping choices, and utilizing time-saving meal prep techniques, individuals with diabetes can streamline their food choices, save time, and ensure they have nutritious meals and snacks readily available. In this section, we'll explore meal planning and preparation tips specifically tailored to the needs of individuals with diabetes.

Creating Balanced Meal Plans

Creating balanced meal plans is key to achieving optimal blood sugar control and supporting overall health and well-being. A balanced meal plan for individuals with diabetes should include a variety of nutrient-dense foods from all food groups, including carbohydrates, proteins, fats, fruits, vegetables, and dairy or dairy alternatives. Here are some tips for creating balanced meal plans:

1. **Portion Control**: Pay attention to portion sizes and aim to include a mix of carbohydrates, proteins, and fats in each meal and snack. Use measuring cups, spoons, and food scales to accurately measure portion sizes and avoid overeating.

2. **Focus on Whole Foods**: Choose whole, minimally processed foods whenever possible, as they tend to be higher in nutrients and lower in added sugars, sodium, and unhealthy fats. Include plenty of fruits, vegetables, whole grains, lean proteins, and healthy fats in your meal plan to provide essential nutrients and support blood sugar control.

3. **Consider the Glycemic Index**: When selecting carbohydrates for your meal plan, consider the glycemic index (GI), which measures how quickly a carbohydrate-containing food raises blood sugar levels. Choose carbohydrates with a lower GI, such as whole grains, legumes, fruits, and non-starchy vegetables, to help stabilize blood sugar levels and promote satiety.

4. **Balance Macronutrients**: Aim to include a balance of carbohydrates, proteins, and fats in each meal and snack to help regulate blood sugar levels and promote fullness. Choose lean sources of protein, healthy fats, and high-fiber carbohydrates to provide sustained energy and support overall health.

5. **Plan Ahead**: Take time to plan your meals and snacks for the week ahead, considering your schedule, preferences, and nutritional needs. Write down a list of meals and snacks, along with any necessary ingredients, to help you stay organized and on track with your meal plan.

By creating balanced meal plans that include a variety of nutrient-dense foods from all food groups, individuals with diabetes can better manage their blood sugar levels, support overall health, and enjoy delicious and satisfying meals.

Smart Grocery Shopping for Diabetics

Smart grocery shopping is essential for individuals with diabetes to ensure they have healthy and nutritious foods on hand to support their dietary needs. Here are some tips for smart grocery shopping for diabetics:

1. **Make a List**: Before heading to the grocery store, make a list of the items you need based on your meal plan and preferred recipes. This will help you stay organized and focused while shopping and prevent impulse purchases of unhealthy foods.

2. **Read Food Labels**: Take time to read food labels and look for products that are lower in added sugars, sodium, and unhealthy fats. Pay attention to serving sizes, carbohydrate content, and ingredients lists to make informed choices that support blood sugar control.

3. **Choose Fresh, Whole Foods**: Fill your grocery cart with a variety of fresh fruits, vegetables, whole grains, lean proteins, and healthy fats. Choose whole, minimally processed foods whenever possible to maximize nutritional

value and minimize added sugars, sodium, and unhealthy fats.

4. **Shop the Perimeter**: Focus on shopping the perimeter of the grocery store, where fresh produce, meats, dairy, and other whole foods are typically located. This will help you avoid the temptation of processed and unhealthy foods that are often found in the inner aisles.

5. **Stock Up on Staples**: Keep your pantry stocked with staple ingredients such as whole grains, beans, canned vegetables, nuts, seeds, and healthy cooking oils. Having these items on hand makes it easier to prepare nutritious meals and snacks at home.

By making a list, reading food labels, choosing fresh, whole foods, shopping the perimeter of the grocery store, and stocking up on staples, individuals with diabetes can make smart choices while grocery shopping and ensure they have a variety of healthy foods on hand to support their dietary needs.

Time-Saving Meal Prep Techniques

Meal prep techniques can help individuals with diabetes save time and make healthy eating more convenient and accessible. By preparing meals and snacks in advance, you can avoid the temptation of unhealthy convenience foods and ensure you have nutritious options readily available. Here are some time-saving meal prep techniques for individuals with diabetes:

1. **Batch Cooking**: Spend some time each week batch cooking staple ingredients such as grains, proteins, and vegetables. Cook large batches of whole grains like brown rice, quinoa, or barley, grill or roast a variety of proteins like chicken, tofu, or fish, and chop up a selection of fresh vegetables. Store these cooked ingredients in separate containers in the refrigerator or freezer, so you can easily assemble meals throughout the week.

2. **Pre-Portion Snacks**: Pre-portioning snacks into individual serving sizes can help prevent overeating and make healthy choices more convenient. Divide snacks like nuts, seeds, trail mix, or cut-up fruits and vegetables into small containers or resealable bags, so you can grab them on the go or pack them in lunches and snacks.

3. **Prepare Overnight Oats**: Overnight oats are a convenient and nutritious breakfast option that can be prepared in advance and customized to suit your tastes. Simply combine rolled oats with milk or yogurt, add your favorite toppings such as fruit, nuts, seeds, or spices, and let it sit in the refrigerator overnight. In the morning, you'll have a delicious and filling breakfast ready to enjoy.

4. **Use Slow Cooker or Instant Pot**: Utilize slow cookers or Instant Pots to prepare hands-off meals that require minimal effort. Simply add ingredients to the pot, set the timer, and

let the appliance do the work while you go about your day. Slow-cooked soups, stews, and chili are hearty and nutritious options that can be enjoyed throughout the week.

5. **Freeze Leftovers**: Don't let leftovers go to waste – instead, freeze them for later use. Portion out leftover meals into individual containers or freezer bags and label them with the date and contents. Frozen leftovers can be easily reheated for quick and convenient meals on busy days.

By incorporating batch cooking, pre-portioning snacks, preparing overnight oats, using slow cookers or Instant Pots, and freezing leftovers, individuals with diabetes can save time and make healthy eating more manageable and accessible. Experiment with different meal prep techniques to find what works best for you and your lifestyle, and make meal planning and preparation a regular part of your routine for better blood sugar control and overall health.

CHAPTER FOUR

Breakfast Recipes

Breakfast is often considered the most important meal of the day, providing essential nutrients and energy to kickstart your morning. For individuals with diabetes, choosing balanced and nutritious breakfast options is particularly crucial for managing blood sugar levels throughout the day. In this section, we'll explore a variety of breakfast recipes designed to provide energy, promote satiety, and support blood sugar control.

Energizing Breakfasts to Start Your Day

Starting your day with an energizing breakfast can set the tone for a productive and satisfying day ahead. Here are some breakfast recipes packed with nutrients and flavor to fuel your morning:

1. Avocado and Egg Breakfast Toast

Ingredients:

- 1 slice of whole grain bread
- 1/2 ripe avocado
- 1 large egg
- Salt and pepper to taste
- Optional toppings: sliced tomatoes, microgreens, hot sauce

Instructions:

1. Toast the whole grain bread until golden brown.

2. Mash the ripe avocado onto the toast and spread it evenly.

3. In a non-stick skillet, fry the egg until the whites are set and the yolk is still runny.

4. Carefully place the fried egg on top of the mashed avocado.

5. Season with salt and pepper to taste.

6. Garnish with optional toppings such as sliced tomatoes, microgreens, or hot sauce.

7. Serve immediately and enjoy!

2. Greek Yogurt Parfait

Ingredients:

- 1/2 cup plain Greek yogurt

- 1/4 cup granola (choose a variety low in added sugars)

- 1/2 cup mixed berries (such as strawberries, blueberries, and raspberries)

- 1 tablespoon chopped nuts or seeds (such as almonds, walnuts, or chia seeds)

- Drizzle of honey or maple syrup (optional)

Instructions:

1. In a serving glass or bowl, layer the Greek yogurt, granola, mixed berries, and chopped nuts or seeds.

2. Repeat the layers until the glass or bowl is filled.

3. Drizzle with honey or maple syrup if desired.

4. Serve immediately and enjoy!

Quick and Healthy Breakfast Options

When you're short on time, quick and healthy breakfast options can help you stay on track with your diabetes management goals. Here are some simple breakfast recipes that can be prepared in minutes:

1. Peanut Butter Banana Smoothie

Ingredients:

- 1 ripe banana

- 1 tablespoon natural peanut butter

- 1/2 cup unsweetened almond milk (or milk of choice)

- 1/2 cup plain Greek yogurt

- Handful of spinach (optional)

- Ice cubes

Instructions:

1. In a blender, combine the ripe banana, peanut butter, almond milk, Greek yogurt, spinach (if using), and ice cubes.

2. Blend until smooth and creamy.

3. Pour into a glass and serve immediately.

2. Veggie Egg Muffins

Ingredients:

- 6 large eggs

- 1/4 cup diced bell peppers

- 1/4 cup diced tomatoes

- 1/4 cup diced onions

- 1/4 cup chopped spinach

- Salt and pepper to taste

- Cooking spray

Instructions:

1. Preheat the oven to 350°F (175°C). Grease a muffin tin with cooking spray.

2. In a mixing bowl, whisk together the eggs, diced bell peppers, tomatoes, onions, chopped spinach, salt, and pepper.

3. Pour the egg mixture evenly into the prepared muffin tin, filling each cup about 3/4 full.

4. Bake in the preheated oven for 20-25 minutes, or until the egg muffins are set and lightly golden brown on top.

5. Remove from the oven and let cool for a few minutes before removing from the muffin tin.

6. Serve warm or at room temperature.

Diabetic-Friendly Smoothies and Breakfast Bowls

Smoothies and breakfast bowls are versatile and customizable options that can be tailored to meet your nutritional needs and preferences. Here are some diabetic-friendly recipes to try:

1. Berry Blast Smoothie Bowl

Ingredients:

- 1 cup frozen mixed berries (such as strawberries, blueberries, and raspberries)

- 1/2 ripe banana

- 1/2 cup plain Greek yogurt

- 1/4 cup unsweetened almond milk (or milk of choice)

- Toppings: sliced strawberries, blueberries, granola, chia seeds, shredded coconut

Instructions:

1. In a blender, combine the frozen mixed berries, ripe banana, Greek yogurt, and almond milk.

2. Blend until smooth and creamy, adding more almond milk if needed to reach your desired consistency.

3. Pour the smoothie into a bowl.

4. Top with sliced strawberries, blueberries, granola, chia seeds, and shredded coconut.

5. Serve immediately with a spoon and enjoy!

2. Green Power Breakfast Smoothie

Ingredients:

- 1 cup unsweetened almond milk (or milk of choice)
- 1/2 ripe avocado
- 1 cup fresh spinach leaves
- 1/2 cup frozen pineapple chunks
- 1/2 small cucumber, peeled and chopped
- Juice of 1/2 lime
- Optional add-ins: protein powder, chia seeds, flaxseed meal

Instructions:

1. In a blender, combine the almond milk, ripe avocado, spinach leaves, frozen pineapple chunks, chopped cucumber, and lime juice.

2. Blend until smooth and creamy.

3. Add any optional add-ins, such as protein powder, chia seeds, or flaxseed meal, and blend again until well combined.

4. Pour into a glass and serve immediately.

These breakfast recipes are designed to provide balanced nutrition, promote satiety, and support blood sugar control for individuals with diabetes. Experiment with different ingredients, flavors, and textures to find combinations that you enjoy and that fit your dietary needs and preferences. With these delicious and nutritious breakfast options, you can start your day off on the right foot and set yourself up for success in managing your diabetes effectively.

CHAPTER FIVE

Lunch Ideas for Diabetics

Lunch is an important meal that provides essential nutrients and energy to sustain you throughout the day. For individuals with diabetes, it's crucial to choose lunch options that help maintain stable blood sugar levels while also providing balanced nutrition. In this section, we'll explore a variety of lunch ideas tailored to the needs of individuals with diabetes, including nutritious salads, flavorful sandwiches and wraps, and warm and satisfying soups.

Nutritious and Delicious Lunch Salads

Salads are versatile, customizable, and packed with nutrients, making them an excellent choice for a healthy and satisfying lunch. Here are some nutritious and delicious salad ideas for individuals with diabetes:

1. Grilled Chicken Caesar Salad

Ingredients:

- 2 cups chopped romaine lettuce

- 4 ounces grilled chicken breast, sliced

- 1/4 cup cherry tomatoes, halved

- 1/4 cup cucumber, sliced

- 2 tablespoons grated Parmesan cheese

- 2 tablespoons Caesar dressing (look for a low-sugar or homemade option)

Instructions:

1. In a large bowl, combine the chopped romaine lettuce, grilled chicken breast slices, cherry tomatoes, and cucumber slices.

2. Sprinkle grated Parmesan cheese over the top of the salad.

3. Drizzle Caesar dressing over the salad and toss to coat evenly.

4. Serve immediately and enjoy!

2. Mediterranean Chickpea Salad

Ingredients:

- 2 cups mixed salad greens

- 1/2 cup cooked chickpeas (canned, rinsed, and drained)

- 1/4 cup diced cucumber

- 1/4 cup diced red bell pepper

- 2 tablespoons crumbled feta cheese

- 2 tablespoons Kalamata olives, pitted and sliced

- 1 tablespoon extra virgin olive oil

- 1 tablespoon balsamic vinegar

- Salt and pepper to taste

Instructions:

1. In a large bowl, combine the mixed salad greens, cooked chickpeas, diced cucumber, diced red bell pepper, crumbled feta cheese, and sliced Kalamata olives.

2. Drizzle extra virgin olive oil and balsamic vinegar over the salad.

3. Season with salt and pepper to taste and toss to coat evenly.

4. Serve immediately and enjoy!

Flavorful Sandwiches and Wraps with a Healthy Twist

Sandwiches and wraps are convenient and portable lunch options that can be customized to suit your tastes and dietary preferences. Here are some flavorful sandwich and wrap ideas with a healthy twist for individuals with diabetes:

1. Turkey and Avocado Wrap

Ingredients:

- 1 whole grain tortilla or wrap

- 2 slices of roasted turkey breast

- 1/4 avocado, sliced

- 1/4 cup baby spinach leaves

- 1 tablespoon hummus

- 1 teaspoon Dijon mustard

Instructions:

1. Lay the whole grain tortilla or wrap flat on a clean surface.

2. Spread hummus and Dijon mustard evenly over the tortilla.

3. Layer sliced roasted turkey breast, avocado slices, and baby spinach leaves on top of the tortilla.

4. Roll up the tortilla tightly to form a wrap.

5. Slice the wrap in half diagonally and serve immediately.

2. Veggie and Hummus Sandwich

Ingredients:

- 2 slices of whole grain bread

- 2 tablespoons hummus

- 1/4 cup sliced cucumbers

- 1/4 cup sliced bell peppers (red, yellow, or orange)

- 1/4 cup shredded carrots

- Handful of mixed salad greens

Instructions:

1. Spread hummus evenly on one slice of whole grain bread.

2. Layer sliced cucumbers, bell peppers, shredded carrots, and mixed salad greens on top of the hummus.

3. Place the second slice of whole grain bread on top to form a sandwich.

4. Cut the sandwich in half diagonally and serve immediately.

Warm and Satisfying Soups for Lunchtime

Soup is a comforting and nourishing option for lunch, especially during colder months. Here are some warm and satisfying soup ideas for individuals with diabetes:

1. Minestrone Soup

Ingredients:

- 1 tablespoon olive oil

- 1/2 cup diced onion

- 1/2 cup diced carrots

- 1/2 cup diced celery

- 2 cloves garlic, minced

- 4 cups low-sodium vegetable broth

- 1 can (14 ounces) diced tomatoes, undrained

- 1 can (15 ounces) kidney beans, rinsed and drained

- 1/2 cup small pasta (such as elbow or ditalini)

- 2 cups chopped spinach

- Salt and pepper to taste

- Grated Parmesan cheese (optional, for serving)

Instructions:

1. In a large pot, heat olive oil over medium heat. Add diced onion, carrots, celery, and minced garlic. Cook, stirring occasionally, until vegetables are tender, about 5-7 minutes.

2. Add low-sodium vegetable broth, diced tomatoes (with their juices), and kidney beans to the pot. Bring to a simmer.

3. Stir in small pasta and chopped spinach. Cook until pasta is tender, about 10 minutes.

4. Season with salt and pepper to taste.

5. Ladle soup into bowls and sprinkle with grated Parmesan cheese, if desired.

6. Serve hot and enjoy!

2. Lentil Vegetable Soup

Ingredients:

- 1 tablespoon olive oil

- 1/2 cup diced onion

- 1/2 cup diced carrots

- 1/2 cup diced celery

- 2 cloves garlic, minced

- 4 cups low-sodium vegetable broth

- 1 cup dried green or brown lentils, rinsed and drained

- 1 can (14 ounces) diced tomatoes, undrained

- 2 cups chopped mixed vegetables (such as zucchini, bell peppers, and green beans)

- 1 teaspoon dried thyme

- Salt and pepper to taste

- Fresh parsley, chopped (optional, for serving)

Instructions:

1. In a large pot, heat olive oil over medium heat. Add diced onion, carrots, celery, and minced garlic. Cook, stirring occasionally, until vegetables are tender, about 5-7 minutes.

2. Add low-sodium vegetable broth, dried lentils, diced tomatoes (with their juices), mixed vegetables, and dried thyme to the pot. Bring to a boil.

3. Reduce heat to low and simmer, covered, until lentils and vegetables are tender, about 20-25 minutes.

4. Season with salt and pepper to taste.

5. Ladle soup into bowls and sprinkle with fresh chopped parsley, if desired.

6. Serve hot and enjoy!

These lunch ideas for individuals with diabetes are designed to provide balanced nutrition, support blood sugar control, and satisfy your taste buds. Experiment with different ingredients, flavors, and textures to create meals that you enjoy and that fit your dietary needs and preferences. With these delicious and nutritious lunch options, you can stay on track with your diabetes management goals and maintain overall health and well-being.

CHAPTER SIX

Dinner Delights

Dinner is an opportunity to unwind, enjoy delicious food, and nourish your body after a busy day. For individuals with diabetes, dinner choices play a crucial role in managing blood sugar levels and supporting overall health. In this section, we'll explore a variety of dinner ideas tailored to the needs of individuals with diabetes, including wholesome one-pot meals for easy dinners, creative ways to incorporate vegetables into main courses, and lean protein options for diabetic-friendly dinners.

Wholesome One-Pot Meals for Easy Dinners

One-pot meals are convenient, time-saving, and perfect for busy weeknights. They require minimal cleanup and can be customized to include a variety of nutritious ingredients. Here are some wholesome one-pot meal ideas for easy dinners:

1. Turkey and Vegetable Stir-Fry

Ingredients:

- 1 tablespoon olive oil

- 1 pound ground turkey

- 2 cups mixed vegetables (such as bell peppers, broccoli, carrots, and snap peas)

- 2 cloves garlic, minced

- 1/4 cup low-sodium soy sauce

- 2 tablespoons hoisin sauce

- Cooked brown rice or quinoa, for serving

Instructions:

1. In a large skillet or wok, heat olive oil over medium-high heat. Add ground turkey and cook until browned, breaking it up with a spoon, about 5-7 minutes.

2. Add mixed vegetables and minced garlic to the skillet. Cook, stirring occasionally, until vegetables are tender-crisp, about 5 minutes.

3. In a small bowl, whisk together low-sodium soy sauce and hoisin sauce. Pour the sauce over the turkey and vegetable mixture in the skillet.

4. Stir to coat evenly and cook for an additional 2-3 minutes.

5. Serve the turkey and vegetable stir-fry over cooked brown rice or quinoa.

6. Garnish with chopped green onions or sesame seeds, if desired.

7. Serve hot and enjoy!

2. Lentil and Vegetable Soup

Ingredients:

- 1 tablespoon olive oil

- 1/2 cup diced onion

- 1/2 cup diced carrots

- 1/2 cup diced celery

- 2 cloves garlic, minced

- 4 cups low-sodium vegetable broth

- 1 cup dried green or brown lentils, rinsed and drained

- 1 can (14 ounces) diced tomatoes, undrained

- 2 cups chopped mixed vegetables (such as zucchini, bell peppers, and spinach)

- 1 teaspoon dried thyme

- Salt and pepper to taste

- Fresh parsley, chopped (optional, for serving)

Instructions:

1. In a large pot, heat olive oil over medium heat. Add diced onion, carrots, celery, and minced garlic. Cook, stirring occasionally, until vegetables are tender, about 5-7 minutes.

2. Add low-sodium vegetable broth, dried lentils, diced tomatoes (with their juices), mixed vegetables, and dried thyme to the pot. Bring to a boil.

3. Reduce heat to low and simmer, covered, until lentils and vegetables are tender, about 20-25 minutes.

4. Season with salt and pepper to taste.

5. Ladle soup into bowls and sprinkle with fresh chopped parsley, if desired.

6. Serve hot and enjoy!

Creative Ways to Incorporate Vegetables into Main Courses

Incorporating vegetables into main courses is a delicious and nutritious way to add flavor, texture, and nutrients to your meals. Here are some creative ways to incorporate vegetables into main courses for individuals with diabetes:

1. Spaghetti Squash with Marinara Sauce

Ingredients:

- 1 medium spaghetti squash

- 2 cups marinara sauce (look for a low-sugar or homemade option)

- 1 tablespoon olive oil

- 2 cloves garlic, minced

- Salt and pepper to taste

- Fresh basil leaves, chopped (optional, for serving)

- Grated Parmesan cheese (optional, for serving)

Instructions:

1. Preheat the oven to 400°F (200°C). Line a baking sheet with parchment paper.

2. Slice the spaghetti squash in half lengthwise and scoop out the seeds and membranes.

3. Drizzle olive oil over the cut sides of the spaghetti squash and season with minced garlic, salt, and pepper.

4. Place the spaghetti squash halves, cut side down, on the prepared baking sheet.

5. Bake in the preheated oven for 40-50 minutes, or until the squash is tender and easily pierced with a fork.

6. Use a fork to scrape the flesh of the spaghetti squash into strands.

7. Divide the spaghetti squash strands among plates and top with marinara sauce.

8. Garnish with chopped fresh basil leaves and grated Parmesan cheese, if desired.

9. Serve hot and enjoy!

2. Stuffed Bell Peppers with Quinoa and Black Beans

Ingredients:

- 4 large bell peppers, any color

- 1 cup cooked quinoa

- 1 cup black beans, cooked or canned (rinsed and drained)

- 1 cup diced tomatoes

- 1/2 cup diced onion

- 1/2 cup diced zucchini

- 1/2 cup corn kernels

- 2 cloves garlic, minced

- 1 teaspoon ground cumin

- 1/2 teaspoon chili powder

- Salt and pepper to taste

- Fresh cilantro leaves, chopped (optional, for serving)

- Avocado slices (optional, for serving)

Instructions:

1. Preheat the oven to 375°F (190°C). Grease a baking dish with cooking spray.

2. Slice the tops off the bell peppers and remove the seeds and membranes.

3. In a large mixing bowl, combine cooked quinoa, black beans, diced tomatoes, diced onion, diced zucchini, corn kernels, minced garlic, ground cumin, chili powder, salt, and pepper.

4. Spoon the quinoa and black bean mixture evenly into the hollowed-out bell peppers.

5. Place the stuffed bell peppers in the prepared baking dish.

6. Cover the baking dish with aluminum foil and bake in the preheated oven for 30-35 minutes, or until the peppers are tender.

7. Remove the foil and bake for an additional 5-10 minutes, or until the filling is heated through and the tops of the peppers are slightly golden brown.

8. Garnish with chopped fresh cilantro leaves and avocado slices, if desired.

9. Serve hot and enjoy!

Lean Protein Options for Diabetic-Friendly Dinners

Incorporating lean protein into your dinners is essential for supporting muscle health, promoting satiety, and maintaining stable blood sugar levels. Here are some lean protein options for diabetic-friendly dinners:

1. Baked Salmon with Lemon and Herbs

Ingredients:

- 4 salmon fillets (about 4-6 ounces each)
- 2 tablespoons olive oil
- 2 tablespoons fresh lemon juice
- 2 cloves garlic, minced
- 1 teaspoon dried thyme
- 1 teaspoon dried rosemary
- Salt and pepper to taste
- Lemon slices, for garnish
- Fresh parsley, chopped, for garnish

Instructions:

1. Preheat the oven to 400°F (200°C). Line a baking sheet with parchment paper.

2. Place the salmon fillets on the prepared baking sheet.

3. In a small bowl, whisk together olive oil, lemon juice, minced garlic, dried thyme, dried rosemary, salt, and pepper.

4. Drizzle the lemon and herb mixture over the salmon fillets, coating them evenly.

5. Place a lemon slice on top of each salmon fillet.

6. Bake in the preheated oven for 12-15 minutes, or until the salmon is cooked through and flakes easily with a fork.

7. Garnish with chopped fresh parsley.

8. Serve hot and enjoy!

2. Grilled Chicken Breast with Roasted Vegetables

Ingredients:

- 4 boneless, skinless chicken breasts

- 2 tablespoons olive oil

- 2 cloves garlic, minced

- 1 teaspoon dried Italian seasoning

- Salt and pepper to taste

- 4 cups mixed vegetables (such as bell peppers, zucchini, cherry tomatoes, and red onion), cut into bite-sized pieces

- Cooking spray

Instructions:

1. Preheat the grill to medium-high heat.

2. In a small bowl, whisk together olive oil, minced garlic, dried Italian seasoning, salt, and pepper.

3. Brush the olive oil mixture over both sides of the chicken breasts.

4. Place the chicken breasts on the grill and cook for 6-8 minutes per side, or until they are cooked through and no longer pink in the center.

5. Meanwhile, place the mixed vegetables on a baking sheet lined with parchment paper. Drizzle with olive oil and season with salt and pepper.

6. Roast the vegetables in the preheated oven at 400°F (200°C) for 15-20 minutes, or until they are tender and lightly browned.

7. Serve the grilled chicken breasts with the roasted vegetables.

8. Enjoy!

These dinner ideas for individuals with diabetes are designed to provide balanced nutrition, support blood sugar control, and satisfy your taste buds. Experiment with different ingredients, flavors, and cooking methods to create meals that you enjoy and that fit your dietary needs and preferences. With these delicious and nutritious dinner options, you can end your day on a high note and maintain overall health and well-being.

CHAPTER SEVEN

Snacks and Appetizers

Snacking and appetizers can be enjoyable and satisfying parts of your day, but for individuals with diabetes, it's important to choose options that help keep blood sugar stable while providing nourishment and flavor. In this section, we'll explore a variety of snack and appetizer ideas tailored to the needs of individuals with diabetes, including nourishing snack ideas to keep blood sugar stable, homemade chips, dips, and salsas, and finger foods and small bites for parties and gatherings.

Nourishing Snack Ideas to Keep Blood Sugar Stable

Snacking can be an important part of managing diabetes, helping to prevent hunger and stabilize blood sugar levels between meals. Here are some nourishing snack ideas to keep blood sugar stable:

1. Greek Yogurt with Berries and Almonds

Ingredients:

- 1/2 cup plain Greek yogurt

- 1/4 cup mixed berries (such as strawberries, blueberries, and raspberries)

- 1 tablespoon sliced almonds

Instructions:

1. In a small bowl, spoon the plain Greek yogurt.

2. Top with mixed berries and sliced almonds.

3. Enjoy this creamy and satisfying snack that provides protein, fiber, and healthy fats to keep you full and satisfied.

2. Apple Slices with Peanut Butter

Ingredients:

- 1 medium apple, sliced

- 2 tablespoons natural peanut butter (or almond butter)

Instructions:

1. Slice the apple into wedges or rounds.

2. Spread peanut butter on each apple slice.

3. Enjoy this classic combination of sweet and savory flavors that provides fiber, protein, and healthy fats to keep you energized throughout the day.

Homemade Chips, Dips, and Salsas

Making your own chips, dips, and salsas at home allows you to control the ingredients and customize flavors to suit your taste preferences. Here are some homemade recipes to try:

1. Baked Sweet Potato Chips

Ingredients:

- 2 medium sweet potatoes, peeled and thinly sliced
- 1 tablespoon olive oil
- 1/2 teaspoon paprika
- 1/2 teaspoon garlic powder
- Salt to taste

Instructions:

1. Preheat the oven to 375°F (190°C). Line a baking sheet with parchment paper.
2. In a large bowl, toss the sweet potato slices with olive oil, paprika, garlic powder, and salt until evenly coated.
3. Arrange the sweet potato slices in a single layer on the prepared baking sheet.
4. Bake in the preheated oven for 15-20 minutes, flipping halfway through, until the chips are golden brown and crispy.
5. Remove from the oven and let cool slightly before serving.
6. Enjoy these crunchy and flavorful sweet potato chips on their own or with your favorite dip or salsa.

2. Homemade Guacamole

Ingredients:

- 2 ripe avocados
- 1/4 cup diced red onion
- 1/4 cup diced tomato
- 1/4 cup chopped cilantro
- 1 clove garlic, minced
- Juice of 1 lime
- Salt and pepper to taste

Instructions:

1. In a medium bowl, mash the ripe avocados with a fork until smooth.

2. Stir in diced red onion, diced tomato, chopped cilantro, minced garlic, lime juice, salt, and pepper until well combined.

3. Taste and adjust seasoning if necessary.

4. Serve the homemade guacamole with baked sweet potato chips or sliced vegetables for a delicious and nutritious snack or appetizer.

Finger Foods and Small Bites for Parties and Gatherings

When hosting or attending parties and gatherings, having finger foods and small bites on hand makes it easy to enjoy delicious snacks without derailing your diabetes management goals. Here are some ideas for finger foods and small bites:

1. Caprese Skewers

Ingredients:

- Cherry tomatoes

- Fresh mozzarella cheese, cubed

- Fresh basil leaves

- Balsamic glaze (store-bought or homemade)

Instructions:

1. Thread one cherry tomato, one cube of fresh mozzarella cheese, and one fresh basil leaf onto a toothpick or small skewer.

2. Arrange the caprese skewers on a serving platter.

3. Drizzle with balsamic glaze just before serving.

4. Enjoy these bite-sized delights that showcase the classic flavors of tomato, mozzarella, and basil.

2. Cucumber and Cream Cheese Bites

Ingredients:

- English cucumber, sliced into rounds

- Cream cheese (regular or low-fat)

- Everything bagel seasoning

Instructions:

1. Spread a thin layer of cream cheese onto each cucumber round.

2. Sprinkle with everything bagel seasoning.

3. Arrange the cucumber and cream cheese bites on a serving platter.

4. Enjoy these refreshing and creamy bites that are perfect for any occasion.

These snack and appetizer ideas for individuals with diabetes are designed to provide nourishment, flavor, and satisfaction while supporting stable blood sugar levels. Whether you're enjoying a snack at home, hosting a gathering, or attending a party, these recipes and ideas will help you make delicious and diabetes-friendly choices that fit your lifestyle and dietary preferences. With these wholesome snacks and appetizers, you can indulge without compromising your health and well-being.

CHAPTER EIGHT

Desserts without Guilt

Desserts are often associated with indulgence and guilty pleasures, but for individuals with diabetes, finding desserts that are both delicious and diabetes-friendly can be a challenge. However, with a little creativity and some smart ingredient swaps, you can enjoy desserts without guilt. In this section, we'll explore a variety of dessert ideas tailored to the needs of individuals with diabetes, including indulgent yet healthy dessert recipes, sugar-free treats for sweet tooth cravings, and fruit-based desserts for a refreshing end to meals.

Indulgent Yet Healthy Dessert Recipes

Indulging in dessert doesn't have to mean sacrificing your health or blood sugar control. With the right ingredients and preparation methods, you can enjoy decadent desserts that are also nutritious and diabetes-friendly. Here are some indulgent yet healthy dessert recipes to try:

1. Dark Chocolate Avocado Mousse

Ingredients:

- 2 ripe avocados

- 1/4 cup unsweetened cocoa powder

- 1/4 cup pure maple syrup or honey

- 1 teaspoon vanilla extract

- Pinch of salt

- Optional toppings: fresh berries, chopped nuts, shredded coconut

Instructions:

1. Scoop the flesh of the ripe avocados into a food processor or blender.

2. Add unsweetened cocoa powder, pure maple syrup or honey, vanilla extract, and a pinch of salt.

3. Blend until smooth and creamy, scraping down the sides as needed.

4. Divide the chocolate avocado mousse into serving bowls or glasses.

5. Chill in the refrigerator for at least 30 minutes to allow the mousse to set.

6. Before serving, garnish with fresh berries, chopped nuts, or shredded coconut if desired.

7. Enjoy this rich and creamy chocolate treat that's packed with heart-healthy fats and antioxidants.

2. Greek Yogurt Berry Parfait

Ingredients:

- 1/2 cup plain Greek yogurt

- 1/4 cup mixed berries (such as strawberries, blueberries, and raspberries)

- 2 tablespoons granola (choose a variety low in added sugars)

- Drizzle of honey or maple syrup (optional)

Instructions:

1. In a serving glass or bowl, layer plain Greek yogurt, mixed berries, and granola.

2. Repeat the layers until the glass or bowl is filled.

3. Drizzle with honey or maple syrup if desired.

4. Serve immediately and enjoy this creamy and crunchy parfait that's high in protein and fiber.

Sugar-Free Treats for Sweet Tooth Cravings

When craving something sweet, opting for sugar-free treats can satisfy your sweet tooth without causing spikes in blood sugar levels. Here are some sugar-free dessert ideas to try:

1. Sugar-Free Chocolate Chip Cookies

Ingredients:

- 1 cup almond flour

- 1/4 cup sugar-free chocolate chips

- 1/4 cup unsweetened applesauce

- 2 tablespoons coconut oil, melted

- 1 teaspoon vanilla extract

- Pinch of salt

Instructions:

1. Preheat the oven to 350°F (175°C). Line a baking sheet with parchment paper.

2. In a mixing bowl, combine almond flour, sugar-free chocolate chips, unsweetened applesauce, melted coconut oil, vanilla extract, and a pinch of salt.

3. Stir until well combined and a dough forms.

4. Scoop tablespoon-sized portions of dough onto the prepared baking sheet, spacing them apart.

5. Flatten each dough ball with the back of a spoon.

6. Bake in the preheated oven for 10-12 minutes, or until the cookies are golden brown around the edges.

7. Remove from the oven and let cool on the baking sheet for 5 minutes before transferring to a wire rack to cool completely.

8. Enjoy these soft and chewy chocolate chip cookies that are free of added sugars.

2. Sugar-Free Berry Chia Seed Jam

Ingredients:

- 2 cups mixed berries (such as strawberries, blueberries, and raspberries)
- 2 tablespoons chia seeds
- 1-2 tablespoons lemon juice
- Stevia or erythritol, to taste

Instructions:

1. In a small saucepan, combine mixed berries and lemon juice over medium heat.
2. Cook, stirring occasionally, until the berries begin to break down and release their juices, about 5-7 minutes.
3. Mash the berries with a fork or potato masher to your desired consistency.
4. Stir in chia seeds and sweetener to taste.
5. Cook for an additional 5-7 minutes, or until the jam thickens.
6. Remove from heat and let cool to room temperature.
7. Transfer the berry chia seed jam to a jar or container and refrigerate until chilled.

8. Enjoy this naturally sweet and flavorful jam on toast, yogurt, or oatmeal.

Fruit-Based Desserts for a Refreshing End to Meals

Incorporating fresh fruits into desserts is a delicious and nutritious way to satisfy your sweet cravings. Here are some fruit-based dessert ideas to try:

1. Grilled Pineapple with Cinnamon

Ingredients:

- 1 pineapple, peeled, cored, and sliced into rings
- 1 teaspoon ground cinnamon
- Optional toppings: Greek yogurt, chopped nuts, honey

Instructions:

1. Preheat the grill or grill pan over medium-high heat.
2. Sprinkle ground cinnamon evenly over both sides of the pineapple rings.
3. Grill the pineapple rings for 2-3 minutes per side, or until grill marks appear and the pineapple is slightly caramelized.
4. Remove from the grill and let cool slightly.
5. Serve the grilled pineapple rings with a dollop of Greek yogurt, chopped nuts, and a drizzle of honey if desired.

6. Enjoy this warm and fragrant dessert that's bursting with natural sweetness.

2. Fruit Salad with Mint-Lime Dressing

Ingredients:

- Assorted fresh fruits (such as strawberries, kiwi, pineapple, mango, and grapes), diced or sliced

- Fresh mint leaves, chopped

- Juice of 1 lime

- Optional: honey or agave nectar, to taste

Instructions:

1. In a large bowl, combine diced or sliced fresh fruits of your choice.

2. In a small bowl, whisk together chopped fresh mint leaves and lime juice.

3. Drizzle the mint-lime dressing over the fruit salad and toss gently to coat.

4. Taste and adjust sweetness with honey or agave nectar if desired.

5. Chill in the refrigerator for at least 30 minutes before serving.

6. Enjoy this refreshing and vibrant fruit salad as a light and healthy dessert option.

These dessert ideas for individuals with diabetes offer delicious alternatives to traditional sweets while still satisfying your cravings and supporting blood sugar control. Whether you're in the mood for something indulgent yet healthy, sugar-free, or fruit-based, these recipes and ideas will help you enjoy desserts without guilt. With a focus on wholesome ingredients and balanced flavors, you can treat yourself to delicious desserts that fit your dietary needs and preferences.

CHAPTER NINE

Beverages and Drinks

Staying hydrated is essential for overall health, and choosing the right beverages can have a significant impact on managing diabetes. In this section, we'll explore a variety of beverage ideas tailored to the needs of individuals with diabetes, including hydrating beverages for optimal health, low-sugar mocktails and refreshing drinks, and coffee and tea creations for diabetic-friendly sipping.

Hydrating Beverages for Optimal Health

Hydration is crucial for supporting various bodily functions and maintaining overall health. Here are some hydrating beverage options that can help keep you hydrated and support your well-being:

1. Infused Water

Infusing water with fresh fruits, vegetables, and herbs adds flavor and nutrients without any added sugars. Here are some infused water ideas to try:

- Cucumber and mint

- Lemon and lime

- Watermelon and basil

- Strawberry and kiwi

- Orange and blueberry

To make infused water, simply add your choice of ingredients to a pitcher of water and let it infuse in the refrigerator for at least 1-2 hours before serving. The longer it sits, the stronger the flavor will be. Enjoy these refreshing infused waters throughout the day to stay hydrated.

2. Coconut Water

Coconut water is naturally hydrating and contains electrolytes such as potassium, making it an excellent choice for replenishing fluids after exercise or on hot days. Look for unsweetened coconut water to avoid added sugars and unnecessary calories. Enjoy coconut water chilled straight from the bottle or use it as a base for smoothies and mocktails.

Low-Sugar Mocktails and Refreshing Drinks

Mocktails are non-alcoholic beverages that offer all the flavor and refreshment of traditional cocktails without the added sugars and alcohol. Here are some low-sugar mocktail ideas to enjoy:

1. Sparkling Berry Lemonade

Ingredients:

- 1/2 cup mixed berries (such as strawberries, blueberries, and raspberries)

- 1 tablespoon freshly squeezed lemon juice

- 1 teaspoon honey or agave nectar (optional)

- Sparkling water

- Ice cubes

- Fresh mint leaves, for garnish

Instructions:

1. In a glass, muddle the mixed berries with freshly squeezed lemon juice and honey or agave nectar (if using).

2. Fill the glass with ice cubes.

3. Top with sparkling water and stir gently to combine.

4. Garnish with fresh mint leaves.

5. Enjoy this refreshing and fruity mocktail that's perfect for any occasion.

2. Ginger-Lime Mojito Mocktail

Ingredients:

- 1 tablespoon freshly squeezed lime juice

- 1 teaspoon honey or agave nectar

- 1/2 teaspoon grated fresh ginger

- Sparkling water

- Ice cubes

- Fresh mint leaves, for garnish

Instructions:

1. In a glass, combine freshly squeezed lime juice, honey or agave nectar, and grated fresh ginger.

2. Fill the glass with ice cubes.

3. Top with sparkling water and stir gently to combine.

4. Garnish with fresh mint leaves.

5. Enjoy this zesty and invigorating mocktail that's bursting with flavor.

Coffee and Tea Creations for Diabetic-Friendly Sipping

Coffee and tea are popular beverages enjoyed by many, and they can be incorporated into a diabetes-friendly diet with some mindful choices. Here are some coffee and tea creations to savor:

1. Iced Green Tea with Lemon and Mint

Ingredients:

- 1 green tea bag

- 1 cup boiling water

- Ice cubes

- Freshly squeezed lemon juice

- Fresh mint leaves

Instructions:

1. Place a green tea bag in a cup and pour boiling water over it.

2. Steep for 3-5 minutes, then remove the tea bag and let the tea cool to room temperature.

3. Once cooled, transfer the tea to a glass filled with ice cubes.

4. Add freshly squeezed lemon juice to taste.

5. Garnish with fresh mint leaves.

6. Enjoy this refreshing and antioxidant-rich iced green tea on a hot day.

2. Cinnamon Vanilla Almond Milk Latte

Ingredients:

- 1 cup unsweetened almond milk

- 1/2 teaspoon ground cinnamon

- 1/2 teaspoon vanilla extract

- Stevia or erythritol, to taste (optional)

- Espresso or strongly brewed coffee

Instructions:

1. In a small saucepan, heat unsweetened almond milk over medium heat until warm but not boiling.

2. Stir in ground cinnamon, vanilla extract, and sweetener if desired.

3. Froth the almond milk using a frother or immersion blender until foamy.

4. Pour espresso or strongly brewed coffee into a mug.

5. Top with frothed almond milk.

6. Sprinkle with a dash of ground cinnamon for garnish.

7. Enjoy this creamy and aromatic almond milk latte as a comforting treat.

These beverage ideas for individuals with diabetes offer delicious alternatives to sugary drinks while providing hydration and enjoyment. Whether you're looking for refreshing mocktails, coffee and tea creations, or hydrating beverages, these recipes and ideas will help you stay hydrated and satisfied while managing your blood sugar levels. With a focus on natural flavors and low-sugar options, you can indulge in delicious drinks without compromising your health and well-being.

CHAPTER TEN

Special Occasion Menus

Special occasions such as parties, celebrations, holidays, and dining out can present challenges for individuals with diabetes. However, with careful planning and thoughtful choices, you can enjoy these events while still managing your blood sugar levels effectively. In this section, we'll explore a variety of special occasion menus tailored to the needs of individuals with diabetes, including hosting diabetic-friendly parties and celebrations, holiday feasts with a health-conscious twist, and dining out strategies for diabetics.

Hosting Diabetic-Friendly Parties and Celebrations

Hosting a party or celebration while managing diabetes requires attention to detail and consideration for the dietary needs of your guests. Here are some tips for hosting diabetic-friendly parties and celebrations:

1. Offer a Variety of Healthy Options

Provide a diverse selection of foods that cater to different dietary preferences and restrictions, including diabetic-friendly options. Incorporate plenty of fruits, vegetables, lean proteins, and whole grains into your menu. Opt for dishes that are baked, grilled, or steamed rather than fried or heavily processed.

2. Limit Sugary Beverages

Instead of serving sugary sodas and cocktails, offer a variety of low-sugar or sugar-free beverages such as infused water, unsweetened iced tea, sparkling water with citrus slices, and sugar-free mocktails. Provide plenty of water to keep guests hydrated throughout the event.

3. Create Balanced Meal Options

Ensure that your menu includes balanced meal options that contain a mix of carbohydrates, proteins, and healthy fats. Offer dishes that are high in fiber and low in added sugars to help stabilize blood sugar levels. Consider serving a variety of salads, grilled meats, roasted vegetables, and whole grain side dishes.

Holiday Feasts with a Health-Conscious Twist

Holiday feasts are often associated with indulgent meals and decadent desserts, but individuals with diabetes can still enjoy these celebrations with some health-conscious adjustments. Here are some tips for preparing holiday feasts with a health-conscious twist:

1. Modify Traditional Recipes

Modify traditional holiday recipes to make them more diabetes-friendly by reducing added sugars, using whole grain flours, and incorporating plenty of fruits and vegetables. Experiment with herbs, spices, and flavorful ingredients to enhance the taste of your dishes without relying on excessive salt or sugar.

2. Serve Lighter Dessert Options

Offer lighter dessert options that are lower in sugar and higher in fiber. Consider serving fruit-based desserts such as baked apples, poached pears, or fruit salads with a dollop of Greek yogurt. You can also experiment with sugar-free or low-sugar dessert recipes that use alternative sweeteners.

3. Encourage Physical Activity

Incorporate physical activity into your holiday celebrations by organizing outdoor games, walks, or other fun activities that promote movement and social interaction. Encourage guests to participate in physical activities before or after the meal to help offset the effects of indulgent holiday foods.

Dining Out Strategies for Diabetics

Dining out can be challenging for individuals with diabetes due to the abundance of high-calorie, high-carbohydrate options available at restaurants. However, with some strategic planning and mindful choices, you can navigate restaurant menus while managing your blood sugar levels effectively. Here are some dining out strategies for diabetics:

1. Research Restaurant Menus in Advance

Before dining out, take the time to research restaurant menus online to identify diabetic-friendly options. Look for dishes that are grilled, baked, or steamed rather than fried or sautéed. Choose dishes that are high in protein, fiber, and healthy fats, and low in added sugars and refined carbohydrates.

2. Make Special Requests

Don't hesitate to make special requests or modifications to your meal to better suit your dietary needs. Ask for dressings and sauces on the side, request substitutions for starchy side dishes with extra vegetables, and inquire about the preparation methods used for menu items. Most restaurants are willing to accommodate special dietary requests.

3. Practice Portion Control

Practice portion control when dining out by ordering smaller portions, sharing dishes with dining companions, or asking for a to-go box to save leftovers for later. Be mindful of portion sizes and listen to your body's hunger and fullness cues to prevent overeating.

By following these special occasion menus and strategies, individuals with diabetes can enjoy parties, celebrations, holidays, and dining out experiences while still managing their blood sugar levels effectively. With a focus on balanced meals, healthy choices, and moderation, you can savor delicious foods and create memorable moments with family and friends without compromising your health and well-being.

The Warrior Diet:

Definition:

The Warrior Diet is an intermittent fasting approach that involves extended periods of fasting followed by short eating windows. Inspired by ancient warrior cultures, this diet encourages individuals to fast for approximately 20 hours each day and consume one large meal during a 4-hour "overeating" window in the evening. During the fasting period, individuals are encouraged to consume small amounts of raw fruits, vegetables, and non-caloric beverages to support hydration and provide minimal energy. The Warrior Diet is believed to promote fat loss, improve metabolic health, and increase mental clarity and focus by aligning eating patterns with natural circadian rhythms.

Ingredients:

- Fasting Period: During the fasting period, individuals consume small amounts of raw fruits, vegetables, and non-caloric beverages such as water, herbal tea, or black coffee.

- Overeating Window: During the overeating window, individuals consume one large meal that includes a variety of nutrient-dense foods such as lean proteins, whole grains, fruits, vegetables, healthy fats, and dairy or dairy alternatives.

Instructions/How to Prepare:

1. Determine fasting and eating windows based on personal preferences, lifestyle, and schedule.

2. Start the day with hydration by drinking water, herbal tea, or black coffee during the fasting period to support overall health and well-being.

3. Consume small amounts of raw fruits and vegetables throughout the fasting period to help manage hunger and provide essential nutrients.

4. Break the fast with a large, nutrient-dense meal during the overeating window, incorporating a variety of foods such as lean proteins, whole grains, fruits, vegetables, healthy fats, and dairy or dairy alternatives.

5. Practice mindful eating during the overeating window, focusing on hunger and fullness cues and savoring each bite of food.

6. Stay hydrated throughout the day by drinking plenty of water and other non-caloric beverages to support hydration and overall health.

7. Experiment with different meal compositions and timing strategies to find what works best for individual preferences and goals.

8. Listen to your body and adjust eating patterns as needed based on hunger, energy levels, and overall well-being.

9. Be patient and flexible, recognizing that intermittent fasting may take time to adapt to and may not be suitable for everyone.

10.   Consult with a healthcare professional or registered dietitian before starting the Warrior Diet, especially if you have underlying health conditions or concerns about fasting.

The Blood Sugar Solution Diet:

Definition:

The Blood Sugar Solution Diet, developed by Dr. Mark Hyman, is a comprehensive approach to managing blood sugar levels and promoting overall health and well-being. It focuses on reducing inflammation, balancing blood sugar, and optimizing metabolism through dietary changes, lifestyle modifications, and targeted supplementation. The diet emphasizes whole, nutrient-dense foods that support stable blood sugar levels, such as non-starchy vegetables, lean proteins, healthy fats, and low-glycemic carbohydrates. It also encourages individuals to eliminate processed foods, refined sugars, artificial additives, and other inflammatory substances from their diet to reduce insulin resistance and improve metabolic function.

Ingredients:

- Whole Foods: Non-starchy vegetables, leafy greens, lean proteins, nuts, seeds, legumes, whole grains, healthy fats, and low-glycemic fruits are emphasized on The Blood Sugar Solution Diet.

- Nutrient-Dense Foods: Foods rich in essential nutrients, vitamins, minerals, and antioxidants are prioritized to support overall health and well-being.

- Elimination of Processed Foods: Processed foods, refined sugars, artificial additives, trans fats, and other inflammatory substances are eliminated or minimized to reduce inflammation and support metabolic health.

- Hydration: Adequate hydration is important on The Blood Sugar Solution Diet, so drinking water, herbal tea, and other non-caloric beverages is encouraged.

Instructions/How to Prepare:

1. Familiarize yourself with the principles of The Blood Sugar Solution Diet, including recommendations for food choices, portion sizes, meal timing, and lifestyle habits.

2. Stock your kitchen with whole, nutrient-dense foods such as non-starchy vegetables, leafy greens, lean proteins, nuts, seeds, legumes, whole grains, healthy fats, and low-glycemic fruits.

3. Plan meals and snacks that prioritize whole foods and balance macronutrients to support stable blood sugar levels and optimize metabolism.

4. Focus on eating a variety of colors, flavors, and textures in meals to ensure a diverse intake of nutrients and promote satiety and enjoyment.

5. Minimize or eliminate processed foods, refined sugars, artificial additives, trans fats, and other inflammatory substances from your diet to reduce inflammation and support metabolic health.

6. Pay attention to portion sizes and practice mindful eating by listening to hunger and fullness cues, eating slowly, and savoring each bite.

7. Stay hydrated by drinking plenty of water throughout the day to support overall health and well-being.

8. Incorporate regular physical activity into your daily routine to enhance metabolic function, support weight management, and promote overall fitness and well-being.

9. Monitor blood sugar levels regularly, especially for individuals with diabetes or insulin resistance, and adjust dietary choices as needed to achieve and maintain optimal blood sugar control.

10.   Consult with a healthcare professional or registered dietitian before starting The Blood Sugar Solution Diet, especially if you have underlying health conditions or concerns about dietary changes.

CHAPTER 11

31 DAY MEAL PLAN

Week 1:

Day 1:

- Breakfast: Spinach and mushroom omelet with whole grain toast.

- Lunch: Grilled chicken salad with mixed greens, cherry tomatoes, and balsamic vinaigrette.

- Dinner: Baked salmon with roasted asparagus and quinoa.

Day 2:

- Breakfast: Greek yogurt parfait with mixed berries and a sprinkle of almonds.

- Lunch: Turkey and avocado wrap with lettuce in a whole wheat tortilla.

- Dinner: Stir-fried tofu with mixed vegetables and brown rice.

Day 3:

- Breakfast: Overnight oats with sliced bananas and chopped walnuts.

- Lunch: Lentil soup with a side of mixed green salad.

- Dinner: Baked chicken breast with roasted Brussels sprouts and sweet potato.

Day 4:

- Breakfast: Smoothie made with spinach, banana, Greek yogurt, and almond milk.
- Lunch: Tuna salad lettuce wraps with cucumber slices.
- Dinner: Grilled sirloin steak with roasted vegetables and quinoa.

Day 5:

- Breakfast: Whole grain toast with mashed avocado and tomato slices.
- Lunch: Quinoa and black bean salad with cherry tomatoes and lime vinaigrette.
- Dinner: Baked cod with roasted zucchini and brown rice.

Day 6:

- Breakfast: Cottage cheese with pineapple chunks and a sprinkle of cinnamon.
- Lunch: Turkey and cheese roll-up with whole wheat tortilla and carrot sticks.
- Dinner: Stir-fried shrimp with bell peppers and snow peas served over cauliflower rice.

Day 7:

- Breakfast: Scrambled eggs with diced tomatoes and spinach.
- Lunch: Greek salad with feta cheese, olives, tomatoes, and Greek dressing.
- Dinner: Beef and vegetable stir-fry with broccoli, carrots, and brown rice.

Week 2:

Day 8:

- Breakfast: Whole grain cereal with low-fat milk and fresh berries.
- Lunch: Hummus and veggie wrap with whole wheat tortilla.
- Dinner: Lentil curry with spinach and quinoa.

Day 9:

- Breakfast: Peanut butter and banana smoothie with spinach and almond milk.
- Lunch: Chicken Caesar salad with romaine lettuce, Parmesan cheese, and Caesar dressing.
- Dinner: Baked tofu with roasted Brussels sprouts and wild rice.

Day 10:

- Breakfast: Yogurt parfait with granola, mixed berries, and honey.

- Lunch: Caprese salad with fresh mozzarella, tomatoes, basil, and balsamic glaze.

- Dinner: Grilled salmon with roasted cauliflower and quinoa.

Day 11:

- Breakfast: Oatmeal with sliced apples and a sprinkle of cinnamon.

- Lunch: Turkey chili with kidney beans and diced tomatoes.

- Dinner: Stuffed bell peppers with ground turkey, quinoa, and tomato sauce.

Day 12:

- Breakfast: Whole grain pancakes with fresh fruit and a drizzle of sugar-free syrup.

- Lunch: Chickpea salad with cucumber, red onion, and lemon vinaigrette.

- Dinner: Lemon garlic roasted chicken with roasted vegetables and barley.

Day 13:

- Breakfast: Chia seed pudding topped with sliced strawberries and almonds.

- Lunch: Turkey and vegetable stir-fry with brown rice.

- Dinner: Baked halibut with steamed green beans and couscous.

Day 14:

- Breakfast: Veggie omelet with mushrooms, bell peppers, and onions.

- Lunch: Greek yogurt chicken salad with grapes and celery.

- Dinner: Beef stew with carrots, potatoes, and onions.

Week 3:

Day 15:

- Breakfast: Scrambled eggs with spinach and diced tomatoes.

- Lunch: Quinoa and roasted vegetable salad with a lemon-tahini dressing.

- Dinner: Grilled shrimp skewers with grilled zucchini and brown rice.

Day 16:

- Breakfast: Whole grain toast with mashed avocado and sliced hard-boiled eggs.

- Lunch: Turkey and avocado lettuce wraps with cucumber slices.

- Dinner: Baked chicken thighs with roasted sweet potatoes and green beans.

Day 17:

- Breakfast: Smoothie made with kale, pineapple, Greek yogurt, and almond milk.
- Lunch: Lentil and vegetable soup with a side of mixed greens.
- Dinner: Baked salmon with steamed asparagus and quinoa pilaf.

Day 18:

- Breakfast: Greek yogurt with sliced strawberries and a sprinkle of granola.
- Lunch: Tuna salad with mixed greens, cherry tomatoes, and balsamic vinaigrette.
- Dinner: Stir-fried tofu with broccoli, bell peppers, and brown rice.

Day 19:

- Breakfast: Overnight oats with sliced bananas and almond butter.
- Lunch: Hummus and vegetable wrap with whole wheat tortilla.

- Dinner: Grilled sirloin steak with roasted Brussels sprouts and quinoa.

Day 20:

- Breakfast: Cottage cheese with sliced peaches and a drizzle of honey.

- Lunch: Chicken Caesar salad with romaine lettuce, Parmesan cheese, and Caesar dressing.

- Dinner: Baked cod with roasted vegetables and wild rice.

Day 21:

- Breakfast: Veggie omelet with mushrooms, bell peppers, and onions.

- Lunch: Greek salad with feta cheese, olives, tomatoes, and Greek dressing.

- Dinner: Beef and broccoli stir-fry with brown rice.

Week 4:

Day 22:

- Breakfast: Whole grain cereal with low-fat milk and fresh berries.

- Lunch: Turkey and cheese roll-up with whole wheat tortilla and carrot sticks.

- Dinner: Lentil curry with spinach and quinoa.

Day 23:

- Breakfast: Peanut butter and banana smoothie with spinach and almond milk.

- Lunch: Caprese salad with fresh mozzarella, tomatoes, basil, and balsamic glaze.

- Dinner: Baked tofu with roasted vegetables and barley.

Day 24:

- Breakfast: Yogurt parfait with granola, mixed berries, and honey.

- Lunch: Chickpea salad with cucumber, red onion, cherry tomatoes, and lemon vinaigrette.

- Dinner: Grilled salmon with roasted cauliflower and quinoa.

Day 25:

- Breakfast: Oatmeal with sliced apples and a sprinkle of cinnamon.

- Lunch: Turkey chili with kidney beans and diced tomatoes.

- Dinner: Stuffed bell peppers with ground turkey, quinoa, and tomato sauce.

Day 26:

- Breakfast: Whole grain pancakes with fresh fruit and a drizzle of sugar-free syrup.

- Lunch: Quinoa and black bean salad with cherry tomatoes and lime vinaigrette.

- Dinner: Baked cod with roasted zucchini and brown rice.

Day 27:

- Breakfast: Smoothie made with spinach, banana, Greek yogurt, and almond milk.

- Lunch: Tuna salad lettuce wraps with cucumber slices.

- Dinner: Grilled sirloin steak with roasted asparagus and quinoa.

Day 28:

- Breakfast: Scrambled eggs with diced bell peppers and onions.

- Lunch: Greek salad with feta cheese, olives, tomatoes, and Greek dressing.

- Dinner: Beef and vegetable stir-fry with broccoli, carrots, and brown rice.

Week 5:

Day 29:

- Breakfast: Greek yogurt parfait with mixed berries and a sprinkle of almonds.

- Lunch: Turkey and avocado wrap with lettuce in a whole wheat tortilla.

- Dinner: Baked salmon with steamed broccoli and quinoa.

Day 30:

- Breakfast: Spinach and feta omelet with whole grain toast.

- Lunch: Grilled chicken salad with mixed greens, cucumbers, and balsamic vinaigrette.

- Dinner: Stir-fried tofu with mixed vegetables and brown rice.

Day 31:

- Breakfast: Overnight oats with sliced bananas and chopped walnuts.

- Lunch: Lentil soup with a side of mixed green salad.

- Dinner: Baked chicken breast with roasted Brussels sprouts and sweet potato.

THE END